SIGNAL DETECTION & MANAGEMENT

www.Pro-career.net

SIGNAL DETECTION

Process

Methods

GVP MODULE IX

Terminology

Structures and Processes

Quality

Operational Aspects

SIGNAL DETECTION

WHO definition: Reported information on a possible causal relationship between an adverse event and a drug, the relationship being unknown or incompletely documented previously.

The CIOMS Working Group VIII (CIOMS, Geneva 2010) definition: A signal is information that arises from one or multiple sources (including observations and experiments), which suggests a new potentially causal association, or a new aspect of a known association, between an intervention and an event or set of related events, either adverse or beneficial, that is judged to be of sufficient likelihood to justify verificatory action

Signal detection (SD) is advanced safety surveillance. The objective of signal detection is to identify adverse events that were earlier considered unexpected or were unknown and appropriately highlight this in the labeling information.

Usually more than a single report is required to generate a signal, depending upon the event and quality of the information available.

Signal detection involves a range of techniques. Data mining is an approach in signal detection that has gained importance due to availability of computed programs. Data mining is carried out on the databases that are available with the sponsor or a regulatory authority. Individual Case Safety Reports from such databases are retrieved and converted into structured format.

Statistical algorithms are applied to this structured dataset to calculate measures of association. If the statistical measure crosses a set threshold, then it is considered to be a signal. Signals are typically generated in drug-event pairs - an adverse event associated with a particular drug. Signals which are significant require further analysis using all available data either to confirm or refute the signal. If this in-depth analysis is non-conclusive, more data may be needed which can be obtained by initiating specific studies such as a post-marketing observational trial.

The detection of early warning signs has certain challenges:

- Adverse drug effects are heterogenous and require meticulous analysis.
- New signals may differ from earlier signals lending to possible confusion.
- Signals are both qualitative and quantitative and both aspects need to be addressed.
- Different types of adverse events require different methods for detection.
- Signal detection should ultimately inform whether risks have changed.

Types of events

Type A: Events related to the pharmaceutical activity of the drug and are dosage dependent.

Type B: Allergic or unpredictable reactions and mostly not dosage dependent. These are seen in a small subset of patients.

Type C: Events that occur due to a disease rather than as an outcome of drug usage.

Pharmacovigilance is mainly able to detect type B and unusual type A events. Analysis of Type C events is complex and poses a challenge.

PROCESS OF SIGNAL DETECTION

Signals are obtained by analysis of reports from spontaneous reports, prescription event monitoring, case-control surveillance, literature information, registries and studies - clinical trials or non-interventional studies

Signals from spontaneous reports may be detected from ICSRs, literature, PBRERs and information from regulatory documents such as variations, renewals, and risk-benefit plans. Poison centers, teratology information services or vaccine surveillance programs also contribute ICSRs in addition to reports from consumers and HCPs.

Active surveillance is based on coordination with healthcare professionals for prescription event monitoring. Creating a network of general practitioners and clinics allows reporting of specified events or events for specified drugs. Signals may arise from studies - interventional and observational, meta-analyses, registries (AED – antiepileptic drug registry, pregnancy registry etc) and literature search.

Strength of evidence in a signal depends on the following factors:

Strength of the association: Are there associated causative factors other than the suspect drug that could impact the signal. How strong is the drug – signal association?

Consistency of the data: Inconsistent data is a hindrance to arrive at a definite conclusion

Exposure response relationship: All angles of the exposure to the drug and occurrence of the event to be analyzed.

Biological plausibility: Is the condition reported medically reasonable or is it erroneous data.

Study findings: Take study findings into consideration

The nature and quality of the data: Are all relevant details reported or is it a scant report. What is the indication for the drug? Is it different in different countries? What is the indication being assessed.

Signal Management Process

- Detection: Identify signals from various sources.
- Validation: Data validation for factual accuracy.
- Prioritization: Signal prioritization.
- Evaluation: In-depth assessment to finally confirm or refute signal.
- Recommendation: Action to be taken.
- Implementation: Implementation of the recommendation.

The focus during review of case reports initially can be on designated medical events (DME) and targeted medical events (TME).

Designated medical events are serious and rare events which have high drug-attributable possibility.

Targeted medical events are events of specific interest with regard to the drug.

Disproportionality-based Signal Detection Methods.

- Empirical Bayes multi-item gamma Poisson shrinker (MGPS)
- Proportional reporting ratio (PRR)

These perform differently with respect to the number and types of signals detected. In a comparative study it was reported that MPGS provides an objective and stable data.

A high-specificity disproportionality method combined with in depth medical analysis is the best way to conduct a quantitative and qualitative assessment.

The FDA has been trying out newer automated and rapid Bayesian data mining techniques to run through MedWatch. The data mining method, the Gamma Poisson Shrinker (GPS) program has now been replaced by the Multi-Item Gamma Poisson Shrinker (MGPS) program.

The MGPS algorithm signal calculates not only for pairs, but also for combinations of drugs.

Hence, events that are more frequent than just the drug – event pair associations are captured. MGPS minimizes random patterns and throws up consistent signals. The MGPS algorithm is also being evaluated to detect drug interactions and to detect differences among subgroups of gender and age. But MGPS cannot differentiate between known associations and new associations.

Signals of disproportionate reporting (SDR).

Statistical methods are particularly useful for analysis of large volume of ICSRs. Statistical methods identify and prioritize the signals. The next step is to analyze the additional factors and conduct an in-depth assessment to finally confirm or refute the signal.

Signals of disproportionate reporting (SDR) require evaluation of case reports, literature information, preclinical, pharmacoepidemiological and study data. Without statistical methods, analysis of such huge volume of data is just not possible.

Systematic Evaluation Of SDR

Signals of disproportionate reporting identified for further evaluation with statistical methods should be medically assessed. False positive results thrown up during statistical analysis have to be rejected. Statistical analysis currently has the disadvantage of not being able to thoroughly evaluate concomitant drug-event pairs and drug-drug interaction. These aspects as well as disease progression or concomitant disease has to be assessed by the medical reviewer. Combination of statistical methods with the classical method of in-depth review is the systematic evaluation of SDRs.

GVP GUIDELINES FOR SIGNAL MANAGEMENT

Guideline on good pharmacovigilance practices for Signal Management (GVP) – Module IX

Based on

1. SCOPE Work Package Signal Management: Best Practice Guide
2. Council for International Organizations of Medical Sciences (CIOMS). Report of CIOMS Working Group VIII on Practical Aspects of Signal Detection in Pharmacovigilance. Geneva: CIOMS; 2010.

Signal: Information arising from one or multiple sources, including observations and experiments, which suggests a new potentially causal association, or a new aspect of a known association between an intervention and an event or set of related events, either adverse or beneficial, that is judged to be of sufficient likelihood to justify verificatory action.

New aspects of a known association may include:

a. Changes in the frequency

b. Changes in gender distribution

c. Changes in age distribution

d. Changes in country distribution

e. Changes in duration, severity or outcome of the adverse reaction.

SIGNAL MANAGEMENT PROCESS

Signal management process: A set of activities performed to determine whether, based on

a. An evaluation of individual case safety reports (ICSRs)
b. Aggregated data from active studies
c. Literature search
d. Other data sources

there are new risks associated with an active substance or a drug or if known risks have changed.

The management process also includes recommendations, decisions, communications and tracking.

The EU signal management process includes:

- Signal detection
- Signal validation
- Signal confirmation
- Signal analysis and prioritization
- Signal assessment and recommendation for action

Signal detection: The process of identifying signals using data from any source.

Signal validation: Evaluating the source data to verify that there is sufficient evidence regarding the existence of a new potentially causal association, or a new aspect of a known association, and therefore justifies further analysis. This should take into consideration the strength of the evidence, the clinical relevance and the previous awareness of the association.

- Validated signal: It can be concluded from the available evidence that there is existence of a new potentially causal association, or a new aspect of a known association, and therefore further analysis of the signal is needed.
- Non-validated signal: When the available information does not have enough evidence regarding the existence of a new potentially causal association, or a new aspect of a known association, and it can be concluded that further analysis of the signal is not needed.

Signal prioritization: Signals with a possible significant patient or public health impact or important shift in the risk-benefit balance of the drug which may need quicker management are prioritized.

Signal assessment: The process of further evaluating a validated signal considering all evidence, to decide whether there are new risks causally associated with the active substance or drug or if known risks have changed. This evaluation can include nonclinical and clinical data and should be as extensive as possible with regards to the sources of information.

Refuted signal: A validated signal after further assessment has been decided to be "false" - a causal association cannot be concluded.

Emerging safety issue

A safety issue considered by a marketing authorization holder to require urgent attention by the regulatory authority because of the potential significant change in the risk-benefit balance of the drug or on the health of the patients or public, and the possible need for immediate regulatory action and communication to patients and healthcare professionals.

Examples

Significant safety issues:

• Identified in ongoing or newly completed studies - an unexpectedly increased rate of lethal or life-threatening events.

• Arising from spontaneous reports or in literature which may lead to considering a contra-indication, a restriction of use, or withdrawal of the drug.

• Related regulatory actions outside the EU such as restriction of use or suspension.

TERMINOLOGY OF THE EU SIGNAL MANAGEMENT PROCESS

Lead Member State: The Member State responsible for monitoring the EudraVigilance database for an active substance or combination of active substances contained in drug authorized in more than one Member State through the national, mutual recognition or decentralized procedures. The lead Member State shall validate and confirm signals on behalf of the other Member States.

If the active substance is authorized in only one Member State, that Member State automatically assumes the responsibilities of the Lead Member State.

PRAC Rapporteur: Rapporteur appointed by the Pharmacovigilance Risk Assessment Committee (PRAC) as part of centralized procedure. Within the EU signal management process, the PRAC Rapporteur is responsible for the confirmation of signals concerning centrally authorized drugs.

Signal confirmation by the PRAC Rapporteur or lead Member State: The process of deciding whether a validated signal entered in the European Pharmacovigilance Issues Tracking Tool (EPITT) requires further analysis and prioritization by the PRAC. This should be done by the PRAC Rapporteur or the lead Member State within 30 days of signal validation. Signal confirmation is not a full assessment of the signal. Signal confirmation kick starts the next step of signal discussion at EU stage and investigation by the PRAC.

Confirmed signal: A validated signal entered in EPITT that requires further analysis and prioritization by the PRAC, according to the PRAC Rapporteur or lead Member State.

Non-confirmed signal: A validated signal entered in EPITT that does not require further analysis and prioritization by the PRAC, according to the PRAC Rapporteur or lead Member State.

Signal analysis and prioritization by the PRAC: The PRAC decides whether a confirmed signal requires further assessment, and if required, under what timelines and procedural process. This is done by evaluating the possible impact of the signal on patients' or public health and the risk-benefit profile of the drug.

Signal assessment by the PRAC: Evaluation of all available data to decide if any regulatory action is required. This is led by a Rapporteur appointed by the PRAC after signal analysis and prioritization.

STRUCTURES AND PROCESSES

Sources of data and information

Signals can be identified from an extensive range of data sources. This includes all scientific information concerning the use of the drug and the outcome of the use - quality, non-clinical and clinical data (including pharmacovigilance and pharmacoepidemiological data).

Sources for signals:

- Spontaneous reports
- Active surveillance studies
- Literature

The periodic monitoring of databases of suspected adverse reactions, which can vary in size is a source of signals. These databases vary in size.

- Marketing authorization holder databases
- National databases,
- EudraVigilance
- WHO Programme for International Drug Monitoring (VigiBase).

This module focuses mainly on signals derived from spontaneous reporting systems. However all sources should be considered during actual signal management.

Signal Detection*

Signal detection process depends on the nature of data, the characteristics (duration of time on market, patient exposure, target population) as well as the type of drug (vaccines and biological medicinal products) which may require different strategies.

Data from all sources should be considered.

Clinical experience and judgement should always be applied.

Signal detection involves a review of ICSRs, statistical analyses, or a combination of both, depending on the size of the data set. When it is not relevant or feasible to assess each individual case (signals from published studies, healthcare record data), assessment of aggregated data should be considered. Guidance on statistical aspects of signal detection should be applied.

The signal detection process should be adequately documented.

Signal Validation*

The following should be considered during signal validation based on the review of ICSR data:

• Prior Awareness

Whether any or all information of the adverse reaction is already included in the summary of product characteristics (SmPC) and package leaflet (PL) of the same drug.

Some signals may only be for a specific drug or a specific formulation. Whether the signal is regarding an adverse reaction already included in the SmPC for other drugs containing the active substance.

Has the signal already been evaluated in the initial application for marketing authorization, the risk management plan (RMP), the periodic safety update report (PSUR) or any other regulatory filing.

• Strength of the evidence.

This depends on

Total number of cases with patient exposure

The number of supportive cases - cases showing a temporal association, positive dechallenge or rechallenge, lack of alternative causes, assessed as potentially related by the reporting healthcare professional and positive results of investigation reports

Cases reported with related terms (other MedDRA terms indicating clinical complications or different stages of the same reaction)

Consistency of the evidence across cases (consistent time to onset, pattern with repeated observations of an association)

Quality of the data and the source

Cases matching internationally agreed case definitions

Dose-reaction relationship

Possible mechanism based on a biological and pharmacological plausibility

Disproportionality of reporting. Any data skewed towards a certain criterion should be investigated.

• Clinical relevance and context

Seriousness and severity of the reaction

Outcome and reversibility of the reaction

More information on an already known adverse reaction - its severity, duration, outcome, incidence or management.

Reactions due to drug-drug interactions

Reactions in vulnerable populations: pregnant women, children, geriatric and patients with pre-existing risk factors

Reactions occurring in different patterns of use (overdose, abuse, misuse, off-label use, medication errors, and falsified products)

• Additional sources of information

This may give more evidence regarding a causal association, or a new aspect of a known association, and may be considered during further assessment of the signal.

These sources are:

Clinical trial data

Findings regarding similar cases in the scientific literature

Information on substances of the same class of medicinal products

Information on the epidemiology of the adverse reaction or the underlying disease

Experimental or non-clinical findings

Databases with larger datasets, if the signal was from national or marketing authorization holder only databases

Healthcare databases that could give information on characteristics of exposed patients and medicine utilization patterns

Information from other regulatory authorities.

Within individual organizations, the signal management process has many phases of subject matter expert discussion. This may result in various decisions A decision tree should be documented as part of the description of the signal management process.

Decision Tree

Signal validation

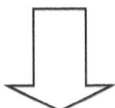

Signal validated?   No - Non-Validated Signal

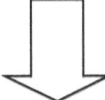

Yes - Validated Signal

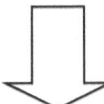

Further assessment with all data

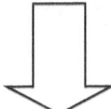

New or changed risk?   No -   Refuted Signal

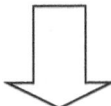

Yes - Confirmed Signal

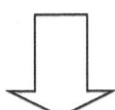

Action changes to the product information
or other risk minimization procedures to be adapted

<u>Signal Prioritization*</u>

Prioritization of signals depends of whether the signals indicate risks that have a significant impact on patient's health, public health or on the risk-benefit balance.

The following aspects influence the prioritization decision:

- Severity, seriousness, outcome and reversibility of the adverse reaction: A more severe and serious reaction is a higher priority.

- The potential for prevention: If it can be prevented then it could move up the priority list.

- Patient exposure and the estimated frequency of the adverse reaction: An increase of both these parameters obviously enhances the priority.

- Patient exposure in vulnerable populations and in populations with different patterns of use: Vulnerable populations need to be handled first.

- Consequences of treatment discontinuation on the disease under treatment and the availability of other therapeutic options

- Expected extent of the regulatory intervention (addition of adverse reactions, warnings, contraindications, additional risk minimization measures, suspension, and revocation): More the regulatory intervention higher is the priority.

- Whether the signal is likely to apply to other substances of the same class of medicinal products.

- Signals that could cause media outcry or public concerns such as adverse events after mass immunization or mass health campaigns may require escalated prioritization.

The timeframe for further management of the signal will depend on the prioritization. Appropriate measures should be considered at any stage if the information available suggests that there could be a risk that requires prevention or minimization in a timely manner. Such measures may be required before a formal assessment of the signal is concluded. Clinical judgement and flexibility should be applied throughout the process.

QUALITY OF SIGNAL MANAGEMENT PROCESS

Signal management is considered a critical process

Any signal management system should be clearly documented to ensure that:

- The system functions in an effective manner.
- The roles and responsibilities are clear and standardized.
- These tasks are done by well qualified and experienced staff.
- There are relevant control measures
- Provision for improvement and enhancement of the system.

A system of quality management should regulate the signal management processes.

This quality system process should be developed, documented and implemented which encompasses analyses, decisions and rationale.

A rationale for the method and periodicity of signal detection activities should be defined.

A tracking system should enable an audit trail of signal management activities, allowing traceability (dates and timeliness) and control of all steps of signal management.

The roles and responsibilities for maintenance of documentation, quality control and review, and for ensuring corrective and preventive action (CAPA) should be assigned.

 Training of staff members in their roles is part of quality initiative.

Description of the signal management process should be in the pharmacovigilance system master file.

Performance indicators should be in the annex to the pharmacovigilance system master file.

A record management system for all documents used for pharmacovigilance activities that ensures the retrievability of those documents as and when needed

Effective record management system ensures traceability of safety concern investigations with regards to decisions, dates and timelines of measures and process activities.

Signal management activities should be audited at regular intervals, including service providers and contractors

Data and document confidentiality, security and validity (including data integrity when transferred between organizations) should be ensured.

Documentation demonstrating compliance with quality systems should be available at any time, including justification and evidence for the steps taken and decisions made.

THE EU NETWORK OPERATIONAL ASPECTS

Responsibilities of the marketing authorization holder in the EU

The marketing authorization holder should continuously monitor the safety of their drugs and inform the authorities of any new information including emerging safety issue that might have an impact on the marketing authorization.

Signals detected via the monitoring of EudraVigilance should be handled in a specific manner.

Signals detected through other sources should be processed as per the signal management system of the marketing authorization holder. These signals should be reported to the relevant EU authorities.

The marketing authorization holder should provide additional information requested by PRAC.

Marketing authorization holders should keep their product information up-to-date considering current scientific knowledge, including the assessments and recommendations made public via the European medicines web-portal

Responsibilities within the EU regulatory network

The regulatory authority of each Member State shall be responsible for monitoring the data originating in that Member State.

Member States and the Agency should validate and prioritize signals they have identified or that have been brought to their notice from any source, including EudraVigilance.

The Agency takes the lead for EudraVigilance monitoring, signal detection and signal validation for active substances contained in at least one centrally authorized product.

Signals validated by the Agency should be confirmed (or not) by the PRAC rapporteur for the specific centrally authorized product.

For active substances only contained in nationally authorized products, Member States take the lead for EudraVigilance monitoring, signal detection, validation and confirmation.

For these substances, Member States may agree to appoint a lead Member State to monitor

EudraVigilance data, detect, validate and confirm signals on behalf of the other Member States.

A co-leader may also be appointed to assist the lead Member State in the fulfilment of its tasks.

The PRAC is responsible for the prioritization and analysis of signals that have been confirmed by the PRAC rapporteur or lead Member State.

The assessment of such confirmed signals is led by the rapporteur appointed by the PRAC at the stage of analysis and prioritization.

Emerging safety issues

When the marketing authorization holder in the EU becomes aware of an emerging safety issue, they should notify it in writing to the Member States authorities where it is approved and to the Agency email "P-PVemerging-safety-issue@ema.europa.eu".

This should be done as quickly as possible and not later than 3 working days after establishing that a validated signal or a safety issue is an emerging safety issue.

In addition, ICSR needs to be submitted as per ICSR submission requirements.

The marketing authorization holder needs to describe the safety issue, the sources of information, any planned or already initiated actions along with their timelines, and should provide documentation available at the time of notification.

Relevant information should be provided to the Agency and national authorities as and when it becomes available.

The national authorities and the Agency should assess the urgency and impact of the emerging issue.

The national authorities and the Agency should agree on steps to be taken and the regulatory procedure to handle the issue. They may have discussions with the Incident Review Network.(European Union Regulatory Incident Management Plan for Medicines for Human Use).

The marketing authorization holder can take the below actions for emerging safety issues with regards to a drug:

- Temporary or permanent cessation
- Suspension of marketing
- Withdrawal from the market
- Request for the withdrawal of a marketing authorization
- Non-application for the renewal of a marketing authorization,

The notification of such action should be to the Agency (withdrawnproducts@ema.europa.eu) and national authorities.

EudraVigilance Monitoring

Member state authorities and the Agency should monitor the EudraVigilance database for new risks or risks that have changed and their impact on the risk-benefit balance. Marketing authorization holders can and should monitor the EudraVigilance database to the extent of their access.

The policy of Access to EudraVigilance data lays down appropriate guidelines.

The member state authorities and the Agency can access all ICSR data.

Marketing authorization holders can access all data elements only of those ICSRs sent by them or from the medical literature monitoring activities done by the Agency.

For other ICSRs, marketing authorization holders can access extended ICSR data elements including case narratives only after signing a confidentiality clause and stating that the ICSR data is required for carrying out pharmacovigilance activities and signal management procedures.

Periodicity of monitoring

Marketing authorization holders, the national authorities and the Agency shall ensure the continuous monitoring of the EudraVigilance database with a frequency proportionate to the identified risk, the potential risks and the need for additional information.

The periodicity of monitoring depends on:

• Duration since authorization.
• Patient exposure.
• Risks documented in the RMP.
• PSUR submission frequency.
• Number of ICSRs.
• Safety in specific situations such as mass health campaigns.

Monitoring of EudraVigilance data should happen at least every 6 months.

A more frequent monitoring is recommended for active substances in the additional monitoring list unless the sole reason for inclusion on the list is for the purpose of a post-authorization safety study (PASS).

EudraVigilance Data Analysis

The selection of drug-event combinations for further review is decided considering

- Number of cases and relevant statistical measures
- Known safety profile
- Clinical relevance (e.g. important medical events)
- Underlying condition
- Patient population
- Previous information and assessments.

The outputs of EudraVigilance monitoring are provided for the active substance or combination of active substances.

Judgment should be applied based on evidence to decide whether a signal is for all or only specific drugs containing an active substance.

For signal validation, a comprehensive analysis of EudraVigilance should be carried out. Marketing authorization holders should consider all ICSR data that are relevant to the safety profile of the drug.

Notifications and Procedures for Signals after EudraVigilance Monitoring

When a marketing authorization holder identifies a new signal during Eudravigilance database monitoring, it should validate and then inform the Agency and national authorities.

Signals should be validated only after a comprehensive analysis of the EudraVigilance information.

Signals validated by the marketing authorization holder should be supported by information from their own database, literature articles and clinical trial data.

A signal should provide new information on a potential causal relationship. Hence, the marketing authorization holder should verify whether the risk may already be presented in the product information of other EU approved drugs containing the active substance. If so, the product information should be modified by applying for variation of the terms of marketing authorization.

The marketing authorisation holder should also consider the information published by the Agency.

Based on their own assessment, the marketing authorization holder can arrive at a conclusion that:

- A signal is refuted
- There is a new or changed risk
- Further analysis is required by the authorities

The conclusion that a signal represents a new or changed risk or that further analysis by the authorities is required is the starting point ('Day 0') of the timelines.

A new or changed risk that requires a change to the terms of the marketing authorization should be the issue or an application for variation.

Further analysis by the authorities may be asked in the case of validated signals that cannot be refuted nor confirmed as new or changed risks by the marketing authorization holder.

Signals requiring further analysis by the authorities maybe reported only in PSURs if the prerequisite condition are met. If not, a standalone signal notification should be submitted

Refuted signals should only be reported in PSURs.

All validated signals requiring urgent attention should be reported as emerging safety issues.

Standalone signal notification

Standalone signal notification is required for signals identified through EudraVigilance monitoring which require further analysis by the authorities.

The form on the European medicines web-site should be filled and sent to the Agency and the Member States authorities where the drug is approved. This should be sent within 30 days after the marketing authorization holder has decided that further analysis by the authorities is required.

Standalone signal notifications are not required in case of signals included within PSURs or variation applications.

Signals refuted by marketing authorization holders should not be sent as standalone signal notifications but should be included in PSURs.

Signal Confirmation*

Within 30 days of a signal validated by the Agency or a Member State, or a standalone signal notification from a marketing authorization holder, the PRAC rapporteur or lead Member State should confirm if the signal should proceed to PRAC analysis and prioritization.

If the signal has been validated by several rapporteurs or lead Member States, confirmation by even one of them will kick start the next step of analysis and prioritization by the PRAC.

A lead Member State or rapporteur can conclude not to confirm a validated signal on the below grounds:

- The information is not enough to arrive at a definite decision or is irrelevant from a medical standpoint.
- It has already been reviewed and the new information is not significant enough.
- It has already been addressed via a different procedure - PSUR or variation - of the drug or other drugs containing the same active substance.

- It has been addressed in the product information of other EU approved drugs with the same active substance.

The reason for not confirming a signal is informed to the Agency and PRAC. This is informed by the Agency to all marketing authorization holders.

Signal Analysis, Prioritization and Assessment by the PRAC.*

When further assessment is required, the PRAC should appoint a rapporteur and define timelines based on the signal prioritization.

The appointed rapporteur should submit an assessment report. The assessment report should include recommendations after considering other PRAC members and the marketing authorization holder's opinions.

The timeframe generally is two months for the submission of additional data by marketing authorization holders and another two months for assessment by the PRAC.

Based on the signal complexity, there may be need for several phases of assessment.

The Agency's website has the timelines for signal assessment. Marketing authorization holders shall work in tandem with the PRAC for the assessment of the signals by providing additional data when required.

Additional information is usually required from marketing authorization holders of the reference medicinal products. The additional information that may be asked may include a cumulative review report (spontaneous reports, clinical trials, literature), with discussion points and conclusion from the marketing authorization holder.

Marketing authorization holders may comment on the rapporteur's preliminary assessment report.

When the PRAC recommends assessment of the signal as per different procedures - PSUR, referral or variation - the process and timelines for that procedure kick in and the signal procedure is closed.

Recommendations on signals from the PRAC.

PRAC recommendations are adopted after prioritization and after each plenary discussion of the signal assessment.

The recommendations may include any or a combination of the below:

The marketing authorization holder should:

- provide additional data for assessment within a signal procedure
- provide a review of additional data of the signal in the following PSUR or submit an ad-hoc PSUR
- update the product information through an application for a variation to the terms of the marketing authorization
- submit an RMP or to update the RMP
- implement additional risk minimization measures such as educational materials or a Direct Healthcare Professional Communication (DHPC)
- should sponsor a post-authorization study and submit the results of that study

The Member States or the Agency should:

- Consider a referral procedure
- Collect further information via the pharmacovigilance non-urgent information system of the EU regulatory network or do additional evaluation.

Other EMA scientific committees or EMA expert groups should be consulted.

An inspection should take place in order to verify that the marketing authorization holder satisfies the pharmacovigilance requirements.

No action is required at this point in time, other than routine pharmacovigilance.

The above are a comprehensive list of recommendations or possible modes of action by PRAC during the signal analysis, prioritization and assessment.

PRAC recommendations for regulatory action such as variation are submitted to the Committee for Medicinal Products for Human Use (CHMP) for endorsement for centrally authorized drugs and to the Co-ordination Group for Mutual Recognition and Decentralised procedures – Human (CMDh) for information in the case of nationally authorized drugs.

The Member States authorities should then action appropriate measures at the national level.

If the Agency or the Member State authority while validating or confirming a signal decides that immediate action is required even prior to the PRAC meeting, it can inform the pharmacovigilance rapid alert system of the EU regulatory network and request discussion on the possibilities to initiate relevant action basis the European Union Regulatory Incident Management Plan.

The PRAC can extend the signal management by allowing it to encompass other active substances of the same class or to other related adverse reactions.

Record management in the European Pharmacovigilance Issues Tracking Tool (EPITT)

The signals validated by the agency as well as those by marketing authorization holders should be entered in the EPITT by the Agency.

Member States should enter the signals validated by them into the EPITT.

The following should be entered:

• Description of the validated signal

• Reason for not confirming for non-confirmed signals

• For confirmed signals: signal assessment report, timetables, PRAC recommendations.

The Agency also enters information on emerging safety issues in the EPITT.

Transparency Of The EU Signal Management Process.

The following information is published by the Agency on the European medicines web-portal:

- PRAC agendas
- PRAC recommendations

For recommendations to update the product information, the agreed wording for the product information is published in all EU official languages, as well as Norwegian and Icelandic. Marketing authorization holders can utilize these translations to update the product information of their drugs

- List of all signals discussed by the PRAC with links to the relevant PRAC minutes
- List of active substances on work-sharing and the lead Member State for monitoring in the EudraVigilance database.
- Outcomes of safety referrals and single assessments of PSURs relevant to signal management.

www.Pro-career.net

- Clinical Research
- Pharmacovigilance
- Drug Safety
- Database
- MedDRA Coding
- Narrative Writing
- Signal Detection

Discussion Forum - Job Portal - Online Library

General Information

A signal often relates to all medicinal products containing the same active substance, including combination products. Certain signals may only be relevant for a particular medicinal product or in a specific indication, strength, pharmaceutical form or route of administration whereas some signals may apply to a whole class of medicinal products.

The continuous monitoring of EudraVigilance is a legal requirement in the EU.

Signals detected through other sources should be reported to EU considering the general obligations of the marketing authorization holder to keep their product information current by variation applications and presenting comprehensive signal information in PSURs.

All Member States are responsible for monitoring EudraVigilance.

Examples of internationally agreed case definitions - Brighton collaboration case definitions for vaccines, RegiSCAR criteria for severe cutaneous adverse reactions.

The marketing authorization holder should coordinate with the Agency and national authorities in the assessment of the emerging safety issue.

For signals identified as emerging safety issues, a standalone signal notification is not required, unless the national authorities and the Agency wish to handle the issue within the EU signal management process, in which case the marketing authorization holder may be requested to provide a standalone signal notification form.

Marketing authorization holders should only communicate as emerging safety issues those safety concerns which meet the definition -- whose urgency and seriousness cannot permit any delay in handling.

New safety information related to quality defects or suspected falsified medicinal products which might influence the evaluation of the benefits and risks which may lead to restriction in supply should not be notified as an emerging safety issue. These should be notified to the Agency (qdefect@ema.europa.eu) or to relevant Member state authorities.

The identification of new risks or changed risks should be based on the detection and analysis of signals.

The frequency of monitoring of EudraVigilance data may vary with the accumulation of knowledge on the risk profile.

Not all disproportionate reporting have to be further investigated as signals and conversely, some drug-event combinations that do not appear as disproportionate reporting may need further investigation.

For signal validation, an analysis of EudraVigilance data should be done along with any previous awareness of the signal on the strength of evidence from the cases (including narrative information) and the clinical relevance.

Record management of the monitoring and analysis of EudraVigilance should be as per the organization's internal procedures

A new or changed risk that requires a change to the terms of the marketing authorization should be the objective of an application for variation of the terms of marketing authorization, unless the marketing authorization holder considers that further analysis by the authorities is needed.

To optimize effectiveness, the system should not transmit less urgent and insignificant information.

The Member State or rapporteur confirming a signal should make a proposal for further management of the signal for the analysis and prioritization by the PRAC.

Standalone signal notifications from marketing authorization holders of nationally authorized drugs with no lead Member State are allocated by the Agency to one of the Member States where the substance is authorized.

The signal assessment report template is on the Agency's website.

Guidance for authorities in Member States is also available in the SCOPE Best Practice Guide on Signal Management.

PRAC recommendations to provide additional data are communicated directly to marketing authorization holders by the Agency.

PRAC recommendations on signals are published on the Agency's website

The fact that a signal is confirmed does not mean that a causal relationship has been established.

www.Pro-career.net

- Clinical Research
- Pharmacovigilance
- Drug Safety
- Database
- MedDRA Coding
- Narrative Writing
- Signal Detection

Discussion Forum - Job Portal - Online Library